CONTENTS

INTRODUCTION

Breast cancer is a formidable adversary that affects millions of lives worldwide. Beyond the medical treatments and therapies available, there is a growing recognition of the significant role that diet plays in both prevention and management of this disease. The saying "you are what you eat" has never held more truth than when it comes to breast cancer. The foods we consume have the potential to either nourish or harm our bodies, and understanding the impact of nutrition on breast health is essential for individuals seeking to take an active role in their well-being.

This book serves as a comprehensive guide to the critical connection between diet and breast cancer. It delves into the latest scientific research, expert insights, and practical strategies to empower readers with the knowledge and tools to make informed dietary choices. From understanding the specific nutrients that promote breast health to discovering powerful anti-cancer foods and incorporating them into daily life, this book provides a roadmap for optimizing nutrition and fostering a supportive environment for prevention, treatment, and recovery.

Within these pages, we will explore the complex interplay between diet and breast cancer, examining how certain foods and dietary patterns can influence the development, progression, and outcomes of the disease. We will unravel the mysteries of phytochemicals, antioxidants, and anti-inflammatory compounds, uncovering their potential to fight cancer and promote overall wellness. Moreover, we will address common dietary misconceptions and debunk myths, allowing readers to navigate the vast landscape of nutritional information with confidence and clarity.

It is important to note that this book is not a substitute for medical advice or treatment. Rather, it is intended as a valuable resource, complementing the care provided by healthcare professionals and offering additional strategies for individuals to take an active role in their breast health. By adopting a holistic approach that combines medical interventions with a well-designed diet, readers can enhance their overall well-being and potentially improve their treatment outcomes.

Throughout this journey, we will discover the power of food as medicine, exploring the potential for dietary interventions to positively impact the prevention, management, and recovery from breast cancer. By harnessing the transformative potential of nutrition, we can empower ourselves and take meaningful steps towards a healthier future. Together, let us embark on this enlightening exploration of the breast cancer diet, with the shared goal of fostering wellness, resilience, and hope.

CHAPTER ONE

Introduction

Understanding breast cancer and its impact

Breast cancer is a complex and multifaceted disease that primarily affects women, but can also occur in men. It is characterized by the uncontrolled growth of abnormal cells in the breast tissue, which can invade surrounding tissues and potentially spread to other parts of the body. The impact of breast cancer is far-reaching, affecting not only the physical health of individuals but also their emotional well-being, relationships, and overall quality of life.

Breast cancer can present with various signs and symptoms, such as the presence of a lump or thickening in the breast, changes in breast size or shape, nipple discharge, or skin changes on the breast. Early detection plays a crucial role in improving outcomes, as it allows for timely intervention and treatment. Regular self-examinations, clinical breast exams, and mammograms are essential for detecting breast cancer at an early stage when it is most treatable.

The role of nutrition in breast cancer prevention and treatment

Nutrition plays a significant role in both the prevention and treatment of breast cancer. A well-balanced diet rich in nutrients can help maintain a healthy body weight, support the immune system, and reduce the risk of cancer development. Here are some key points to consider regarding the role of nutrition:

- Healthy weight management: Maintaining a healthy weight through a balanced diet and regular physical activity is crucial in reducing the risk of breast cancer. Excess body weight, especially after menopause, has been linked to an increased risk of developing breast cancer. A diet rich in fruits, vegetables, whole grains, and lean proteins, while limiting processed foods and sugary beverages, can aid in weight management.
- Phytochemicals and antioxidants: Certain foods, such as berries, cruciferous vegetables (broccoli, cauliflower, Brussels sprouts), and green tea, contain phytochemicals and antioxidants that have been shown to have anti-cancer properties. These compounds can help protect cells from damage, reduce inflammation, and support

overall health.

- Omega-3 fatty acids: Including sources of omega-3 fatty acids, such as fatty fish (salmon, sardines), flaxseeds, and walnuts, in the diet can be beneficial. Omega-3 fatty acids have anti-inflammatory properties and may help reduce the risk of breast cancer.

- Calcium and vitamin D: Adequate intake of calcium and vitamin D is important for overall bone health and may also play a role in reducing the risk of breast cancer. Good sources of calcium include dairy products, leafy green vegetables, and fortified foods. Vitamin D can be obtained through sunlight exposure and certain foods like fatty fish and fortified dairy products.

Goals and benefits of a breast cancer diet

Adopting a breast cancer diet can offer several goals and benefits for individuals facing breast cancer or aiming for prevention. Here are some key points to consider:

- Supporting overall health: A breast cancer diet emphasizes the consumption of nutrient-dense foods, which can support overall health and well-being. It provides essential vitamins, minerals, antioxidants, and phytochemicals that help strengthen the immune system and promote optimal functioning of the body.

- Reducing cancer recurrence risk: Studies suggest that certain dietary patterns, such as the Mediterranean diet, may be associated with a lower risk of breast cancer recurrence. These diets typically include abundant fruits, vegetables, whole grains, lean proteins, and healthy fats while limiting processed foods and saturated fats.

- Managing treatment side effects: A breast cancer diet can help manage the side effects of treatment, such as fatigue, nausea, and weight changes. Consuming small, frequent meals that are easily digestible, staying hydrated, and incorporating anti-inflammatory foods can be beneficial.

- Emotional well-being and empowerment: Nurturing one's body through a breast cancer diet can contribute to a sense of empowerment and control over one's health. It can enhance emotional well-being and provide individuals with a proactive approach to their cancer journey.

In conclusion, understanding breast cancer and its impact is essential for individuals and society as a whole. Nutrition plays a vital role in both the prevention and treatment of breast cancer, offering numerous benefits. By adopting a breast cancer diet, individuals can support their overall health, reduce the risk of recurrence, manage treatment side effects, and experience a sense of empowerment. Remember, knowledge is power, and making informed choices can have a profound impact on the journey through breast cancer.

Fundamentals of a Breast Cancer Diet

Key Nutrients for Breast Health

Breast health is an essential aspect of overall well-being for women. Consuming a balanced diet that includes key nutrients can help support breast health and reduce the risk of breast cancer. In this section, we will explore some of the important nutrients that play a crucial role in maintaining breast health.

1 Antioxidants and Phytochemicals

Antioxidants and phytochemicals are compounds found in various fruits, vegetables, and plants that have been associated with numerous health benefits, including breast health. These compounds help protect the body's cells from damage caused by harmful free radicals. Free radicals can lead to oxidative stress, which has been linked to an increased risk of cancer.

Foods rich in antioxidants and phytochemicals include berries, such as blueberries, strawberries, and raspberries, as well as leafy greens like spinach and kale. Additionally, tomatoes, carrots, and citrus fruits like oranges and lemons are excellent sources. Incorporating these foods into your diet can provide a wide range of antioxidants and phytochemicals to support breast health.

.2 Omega-3 Fatty Acids

Omega-3 fatty acids are a type of polyunsaturated fat that is known for its anti-inflammatory properties. These healthy fats are essential for maintaining overall health, including breast health. Studies have suggested that omega-3 fatty acids may help reduce the risk of breast cancer and improve treatment outcomes.

Good sources of omega-3 fatty acids include fatty fish like salmon, mackerel, and sardines. For those who prefer plant-based options, flaxseeds, chia seeds, and walnuts are excellent choices. Adding these foods to your diet can help ensure an adequate intake of omega-3 fatty acids and promote breast health.

Fiber

Fiber is an important nutrient that aids in digestion and supports overall health. It plays a vital role in maintaining a healthy weight, which is crucial for reducing the risk of breast cancer. High-fiber foods help regulate blood sugar levels and promote satiety, preventing overeating and weight gain.

Whole grains, such as brown rice, quinoa, and whole wheat bread, are excellent sources of fiber. Additionally, legumes like lentils, chickpeas, and black beans are rich in fiber. By incorporating these foods into your diet, you can increase your fiber intake and support breast health.

.4 Vitamins and Minerals

Vitamins and minerals are essential for maintaining optimal health, and certain ones have been linked to breast health. Vitamin D, for example, plays a crucial role in regulating cell growth and division, and a deficiency in this vitamin has been associated with an increased risk of breast cancer. Good sources of vitamin D include fatty fish, fortified dairy products, and exposure to sunlight.

Another important nutrient is calcium, which is essential for maintaining strong bones and may have a protective effect against breast cancer. Dairy products like milk, yogurt, and cheese are rich in calcium, but if you prefer non-dairy options, calcium can also be found in foods like broccoli, almonds, and tofu.

Incorporating a variety of fruits, vegetables, whole grains, and lean proteins into your diet can provide you with a wide range of vitamins and minerals to support breast health.

Foods to Emphasize in a Breast Cancer Diet

While a healthy and balanced diet is crucial for overall health, certain foods are particularly beneficial for breast health and may help reduce the risk of breast cancer. Let's explore some of these foods in detail.

Cruciferous Vegetables

Cruciferous vegetables are a group of vegetables that include broccoli, cauliflower, Brussels sprouts, kale, and cabbage. These vegetables are rich in antioxidants, vitamins, minerals, and fiber. They also contain compounds called glucosinolates, which have been shown to have anti-cancer properties, including breast cancer.

Incorporating cruciferous vegetables into your diet can be as simple as steaming them as a side dish or adding them to stir-fries and salads. They provide a refreshing crunch and a range of nutrients to support breast health.

Berries and Other Colorful Fruits

Berries, such as strawberries, blueberries, and raspberries, are not only delicious but also packed with antioxidants and phytochemicals. These vibrant fruits contain compounds that help reduce inflammation and protect against cell damage, potentially reducing the risk of breast cancer.

In addition to berries, other colorful fruits like oranges, grapes, and pomegranates are also beneficial for breast health. Including a variety of colorful fruits in your diet can provide a wide array of nutrients and contribute to overall well-being.

Whole Grains and Legumes

Whole grains, such as oats, brown rice, and whole wheat bread, are excellent sources of fiber, vitamins, and minerals. They provide sustained energy and help regulate blood sugar levels, which is important for maintaining a healthy weight.

Legumes, including lentils, chickpeas, and black beans, are also rich in fiber and protein. They are a great alternative to animal-based proteins and can be incorporated into various dishes, such as soups, salads, and stews.

By including whole grains and legumes in your diet, you can enhance your nutrient intake and promote breast health.

Healthy Fats and Oils

Healthy fats and oils are an important part of a balanced diet and can be beneficial for breast health. Foods like avocados, olive oil, and nuts are rich in monounsaturated fats, which have been associated with a reduced risk of breast cancer.

Avocado can be enjoyed in salads, sandwiches, or even as a creamy spread. Olive oil can be used as a dressing for salads or as a cooking oil for sautéing vegetables. Nuts make for a convenient and nutritious snack option.

Including these healthy fats and oils in your diet can help support breast health and provide a range of other health benefits.

Lean Proteins

Lean proteins are essential for maintaining and repairing

body tissues. Good sources of lean proteins include poultry, fish, tofu, and legumes. These protein-rich foods provide important amino acids and are lower in saturated fats compared to red meats.

Incorporating lean proteins into your meals can help maintain a balanced diet and support overall health, including breast health.

By emphasizing these foods in your diet, you can promote breast health and reduce the risk of breast cancer. However, it's important to remember that a healthy diet is just one aspect of maintaining breast health. Regular exercise, maintaining a healthy weight, and avoiding harmful habits like smoking and excessive alcohol consumption are also vital for overall well-being and breast health.

Foods to Limit or Avoid in a Breast Cancer Diet

While emphasizing nutritious foods, it's essential to limit or avoid certain foods that may negatively impact breast health.

Processed and Red Meats

Processed meats, such as bacon, sausages, and deli meats,

are often high in saturated fats, sodium, and preservatives. Regular consumption of processed meats has been linked to an increased risk of breast cancer. Red meats, such as beef, lamb, and pork, should also be consumed in moderation as they contain saturated fats that can contribute to inflammation and other health issues. Opting for leaner protein sources, as mentioned earlier, is a healthier choice for breast health.

Sugary Foods and Beverages

High intake of sugary foods and beverages can lead to weight gain and obesity, which is associated with an increased risk of breast cancer. These items, including soda, candy, desserts, and sugary cereals, provide empty calories and little nutritional value. Instead, satisfy your sweet tooth with natural sweeteners like fresh fruits or opt for healthier alternatives like dark chocolate.

Refined Grains and Flours

Refined grains and flours have undergone processing, stripping them of their fiber and nutrients. Examples of refined grains include white bread, white rice, and refined pasta. These foods can cause spikes in blood sugar levels and have been associated with an increased risk of breast cancer. Instead, choose whole grain alternatives like whole wheat bread, brown rice, and whole wheat pasta, which provide more fiber and essential nutrients.

High-Fat Dairy Products

High-fat dairy products, such as whole milk, cheese, and butter, contain saturated fats that can contribute to inflammation and negatively impact breast health. Opting for low-fat or non-fat dairy options, such as skim milk, reduced-fat cheese, or yogurt, is a healthier choice. Alternatively, consider plant-based milk alternatives like almond milk, soy milk, or oat milk.

Alcohol

Alcohol consumption has been linked to an increased risk of breast cancer. It's recommended to limit alcohol intake or avoid it altogether. If you choose to drink alcohol, do so in moderation. The American Cancer Society suggests that women should limit themselves to one alcoholic beverage per day.

By being mindful of your food choices and incorporating a balanced and nutritious diet, you can promote breast health and reduce the risk of breast cancer. Remember to consult with a healthcare professional or a registered dietitian for personalized guidance on maintaining a healthy diet for breast health.

In conclusion, focusing on key nutrients such as antioxidants, phytochemicals, omega-3 fatty acids, fiber, vitamins, and minerals can support breast health. Emphasizing foods like cruciferous vegetables, berries, whole grains, legumes, healthy fats, and lean proteins can provide the necessary nutrients for optimal breast health. Additionally, limiting or avoiding processed and red meats, sugary foods and beverages, refined grains and flours, high-fat dairy products, and alcohol can help reduce the risk of breast cancer and support overall breast health.

Meal Planning for Breast Cancer Recovery

Establishing a Healthy Eating Pattern

Establishing a healthy eating pattern is essential for maintaining overall well-being, including breast health. By focusing on balancing macronutrients, practicing portion control, and paying attention to meal timing and frequency, you can create a nutritious and sustainable eating plan.

- **Balancing Macronutrients:** Balancing macronutrients involves incorporating a proper ratio of carbohydrates, proteins, and fats into your diet. Carbohydrates provide energy, while proteins support cell repair and growth, and fats aid in nutrient absorption and hormone regulation. Aim to include a variety of whole grains, lean proteins, healthy fats (such as avocados, nuts, and olive oil), and plenty of fruits and vegetables in your meals. This balanced approach ensures that you obtain essential nutrients and maintain stable energy levels throughout the day.
- Portion Control: Portion control is crucial for maintaining a healthy weight and avoiding overeating. It involves being mindful of the quantity of food you consume at each meal. Use smaller plates, bowls, and cups to help control portion sizes visually. Additionally, listen to your body's hunger and fullness cues to avoid unnecessary overeating. Including a variety of nutrient-dense foods in appropriate portions can help support optimal breast health.
- Meal Timing and Frequency: Meal timing and frequency play a role in stabilizing blood sugar levels, promoting digestion, and maintaining energy levels. Aim to have regular meals throughout the day, including breakfast, lunch, dinner, and a few healthy snacks in between, if needed. This approach can help prevent excessive hunger and overeating. Additionally, try to eat

meals at consistent times each day to establish a routine that supports your body's natural rhythms.

Sample Meal Plans for Different Stages of Breast Cancer Treatment

During different stages of breast cancer treatment, the nutritional needs of individuals may vary. Here are sample meal plans for three specific stages: pre-surgery, during chemotherapy or radiation, and post-treatment. It's important to note that these are general meal plans, and individual needs may vary. Consulting with a healthcare professional or registered dietitian for personalized guidance is recommended.

Pre-Surgery Meal Plan

Before undergoing breast cancer surgery, focusing on nourishing your body with a well-balanced diet is crucial. Consider the following sample meal plan:

- Breakfast: A bowl of oatmeal topped with berries and a sprinkle of nuts, along with a cup of green tea.
- Snack: Greek yogurt with sliced cucumbers.
- Lunch: Grilled chicken breast salad with

mixed greens, cherry tomatoes, avocado, and a vinaigrette dressing.
- Snack: Carrot sticks with hummus.
- Dinner: Baked salmon with roasted vegetables (such as broccoli, bell peppers, and carrots) and quinoa.
- Evening Snack: A small handful of almonds and a piece of fruit.

During Chemotherapy or Radiation Meal Plan

During chemotherapy or radiation treatment, it's essential to focus on maintaining adequate nutrition and managing treatment-related side effects. Consider the following sample meal plan:

- Breakfast: Scrambled eggs with spinach and mushrooms, whole grain toast, and a cup of herbal tea.
- Snack: A smoothie made with mixed berries, spinach, almond milk, and a scoop of protein powder.
- Lunch: Quinoa salad with grilled chicken, mixed vegetables, and a lemon-tahini dressing.
- Snack: Whole grain crackers with hummus.
- Dinner: Baked cod with steamed broccoli and brown rice.
- Evening Snack: A cup of herbal tea and a small piece of dark chocolate.

Post-Treatment Meal Plan

After completing breast cancer treatment, focusing on

nourishing foods to support recovery and overall well-being is crucial. Consider the following sample meal plan:

- Breakfast: Overnight oats made with almond milk, chia seeds, and mixed berries.
- Snack: A handful of trail mix with dried fruits and nuts.
- Lunch: Grilled vegetable wrap with hummus, served with a side salad.
- Snack: Sliced apple with almond butter.
- Dinner: Baked chicken breast with roasted sweet potatoes and steamed asparagus.
- Evening Snack: Greek yogurt with a drizzle of honey and sliced almonds.

Remember, these sample meal plans are just examples, and individual preferences and dietary restrictions should be considered. It's essential to work with a healthcare professional or registered dietitian to develop a personalized meal plan that meets your specific needs during each stage of breast cancer treatment.

Adapting the Breast Cancer Diet for Different Scenarios

Breast Cancer Prevention Strategies

Prevention plays a vital role in reducing the risk of breast cancer. Implementing certain strategies, including dietary modifications and lifestyle factors, can help lower the chances of developing breast cancer.

Dietary Modifications for High-Risk Individuals

For individuals at high risk of breast cancer, making specific dietary modifications can be beneficial. It is recommended to:

- Increase intake of fruits and vegetables: These foods contain antioxidants and phytochemicals that help protect against cancer.
- Choose whole grains: Whole grains provide fiber, vitamins, and minerals that contribute to overall health and reduce the risk of breast cancer.
- Include lean proteins: Opt for lean sources of protein such as fish, poultry, legumes, and tofu, while limiting consumption of processed and red meats.
- Limit alcohol intake: Excessive alcohol consumption has been associated with an increased risk of breast cancer. It's advisable to limit alcohol or avoid it altogether.

Lifestyle Factors for Breast Cancer Prevention

In addition to dietary modifications, certain lifestyle factors can contribute to breast cancer prevention:

- Maintain a healthy weight: Obesity and excess body fat have been linked to an increased risk of breast cancer. Aim to achieve and maintain a healthy weight through a balanced diet and regular physical activity.

- Engage in regular exercise: Regular physical activity has been shown to lower the risk of breast cancer. Strive for at least 150 minutes of moderate-intensity exercise or 75 minutes of vigorous exercise each week.
- Avoid smoking: Smoking has been associated with an increased risk of various cancers, including breast cancer. Quitting smoking is essential for overall health and cancer prevention.
- Get regular screenings: Early detection is crucial in the successful treatment of breast cancer. Follow recommended guidelines for mammograms and other screenings based on age and risk factors.

The Breast Cancer Diet During Menopause

Menopause is a significant life stage for women, and hormonal changes during this time can impact breast health. The following dietary considerations are important during menopause:

- Addressing Hormonal Changes Through Diet: During menopause, estrogen levels decline. Incorporating foods rich in phytoestrogens, such as soybeans, flaxseeds, and legumes, may help alleviate symptoms and support hormonal balance. These plant-based compounds have estrogen-like effects in the body and can help

> manage menopausal symptoms.

- Foods to Support Bone Health: Estrogen plays a crucial role in maintaining bone density, and its decline during menopause can increase the risk of osteoporosis. To support bone health, include calcium-rich foods such as dairy products, leafy greens, and fortified plant-based milk. Vitamin D, found in fatty fish, egg yolks, and sunlight exposure, aids in calcium absorption and is important for bone health as well.

Long-Term Dietary Considerations for Survivors

After breast cancer treatment, long-term dietary considerations are essential for survivors to support overall health and well-being. Some key aspects to focus on include:

- Managing Long-Term Side Effects Through Nutrition: Breast cancer treatment may lead to long-term side effects such as fatigue, weight changes, and digestive issues. Eating a well-balanced diet with an emphasis on nutrient-dense foods can help manage these side effects. Including a variety of fruits, vegetables, whole grains, lean proteins, and healthy fats provides the necessary nutrients for recovery and helps support the body's healing process.
- Supporting Overall Health and Well-being: A healthy lifestyle is crucial for long-term breast

cancer survivors. Adopting habits such as regular physical activity, stress management techniques, and adequate sleep can contribute to overall health and well-being. Additionally, maintaining a nutritious diet with a focus on whole foods, hydration, and moderation in alcohol consumption can help support optimal health as a breast cancer survivor.

In conclusion, breast cancer prevention strategies involve implementing dietary modifications and adopting a healthy lifestyle. High-risk individuals should consider dietary changes, such as increasing fruit and vegetable intake, choosing whole grains, including lean proteins, and limiting alcohol consumption. Lifestyle factors like maintaining a healthy weight, engaging in regular exercise, avoiding smoking, and undergoing regular screenings are essential for prevention. During menopause, addressing hormonal changes through diet and focusing on bone health are important. Long-term dietary considerations for breast cancer survivors involve managing side effects through nutrition and supporting overall health and well-being through a balanced diet and healthy lifestyle choices.

Conclusion and Final Thoughts

Recap of Key Takeaways

Throughout this discussion on breast health and the breast cancer diet, several key takeaways can be summarized:

- Key nutrients for breast health include antioxidants, phytochemicals, omega-3 fatty acids, fiber, vitamins, and minerals.
- Emphasize a variety of cruciferous vegetables, berries, whole grains, legumes, healthy fats, and lean proteins in your diet to support breast health.
- Limit or avoid processed and red meats, sugary foods and beverages, refined grains and flours, high-fat dairy products, and alcohol to reduce the risk of breast cancer.
- Establish a healthy eating pattern by balancing macronutrients, practicing portion control, and paying attention to meal timing and frequency.
- Sample meal plans for different stages of breast cancer treatment can provide guidance, but individualized recommendations from healthcare professionals or registered dietitians are crucial.
- Breast cancer prevention strategies involve dietary modifications for high-risk individuals, lifestyle factors like maintaining a healthy weight and engaging in regular exercise, and regular screenings for early detection.
- During menopause, addressing hormonal changes through diet and supporting bone health are important considerations.
- Long-term dietary considerations for breast cancer survivors involve managing side effects through nutrition and supporting overall health

and well-being.

Empowering Readers with Knowledge and Tools for a Healthy Lifestyle

Understanding the impact of nutrition and lifestyle on breast health empowers readers to make informed decisions and take control of their well-being. By incorporating the knowledge gained from this discussion into their lives, individuals can make positive changes to support breast health and reduce the risk of breast cancer.

It's essential to recognize that each person's journey is unique, and consulting with healthcare professionals, such as doctors and registered dietitians, can provide personalized guidance and support. They can help develop tailored strategies and meal plans that meet individual needs and address specific concerns.

Additionally, readers can explore resources and tools available online and in their communities to further enhance their understanding of breast health, healthy eating, and lifestyle practices. Education, support groups, and online communities can offer valuable insights, tips, and encouragement for maintaining a healthy lifestyle.

Encouragement for Embracing a Breast Cancer Diet as Part of the Healing Journey

For individuals on a breast cancer journey, adopting a breast cancer diet can be a powerful tool in the healing process. By nourishing the body with nutrient-dense foods, making conscious choices, and embracing a healthy lifestyle, individuals can support their overall well-being and enhance their quality of life.

It's important to remember that the breast cancer diet is not a restrictive or temporary measure, but rather a long-term commitment to wellness. It's a way of embracing a nourishing and balanced approach to eating that can benefit not only breast health but also overall health.

Every step taken towards a healthier lifestyle is a step towards healing and resilience. By prioritizing self-care, making positive changes, and seeking support, individuals can embrace the breast cancer diet as part of their healing journey and empower themselves to live a life of vitality and well-being.

In conclusion, by implementing the key takeaways from

this discussion, readers can empower themselves with knowledge and tools for a healthy lifestyle. Embracing a breast cancer diet as part of the healing journey is a powerful way to support breast health, reduce the risk of breast cancer, and enhance overall well-being. Remember, small changes can make a big difference, and with determination, support, and self-care, individuals can embark on a path of optimal health and healing.

CHAPTER TWO

Grilled Salmon with Steamed Broccoli

Description: This mouthwatering dish features tender grilled salmon fillets paired with vibrant steamed broccoli. It's a perfect combination of flavors and textures that will satisfy your taste buds and nourish your body.

Ingredients:

- 2 salmon fillets
- 2 cups broccoli florets
- 2 tablespoons olive oil
- Salt and pepper to taste
- Lemon wedges for garnish

Instructions:

- Preheat the grill to medium-high heat.
- Season the salmon fillets with salt and pepper on both sides.
- Brush the grill grates with olive oil to prevent sticking.
- Place the salmon fillets on the grill, skin side down. Cook for about 4-5 minutes per side, or until the salmon is cooked through and flakes easily with a fork.
- While the salmon is grilling, steam the broccoli florets until tender, about 5-7 minutes.

- Remove the salmon from the grill and let it rest for a few minutes.
- Serve the grilled salmon alongside the steamed broccoli.
- Garnish with lemon wedges for an extra burst of freshness.

Nutritional Information:

Calories: 300

Protein: 30g

Fat: 18g

Carbohydrates: 8g

Fiber: 4g

Quinoa and Vegetable Stir-Fry

Description: This vibrant and nutritious stir-fry combines fluffy quinoa with a colorful medley of vegetables. It's a quick and easy vegetarian dish that is packed with flavor and provides a good balance of protein, carbs, and fiber.

Ingredients:

- 1 cup cooked quinoa
- 1 bell pepper, sliced
- 1 zucchini, sliced
- 1 carrot, julienned

- 1 cup broccoli florets
- 2 tablespoons soy sauce
- 1 tablespoon sesame oil
- 1 tablespoon olive oil
- 2 cloves garlic, minced
- 1 teaspoon ginger, grated
- Salt and pepper to taste
- Sesame seeds for garnish

Instructions:

- Heat olive oil in a large skillet or wok over medium heat.
- Add the minced garlic and grated ginger, and sauté for 1-2 minutes until fragrant.
- Add the sliced bell pepper, zucchini, carrot, and broccoli florets to the skillet. Stir-fry for 4-5 minutes until the vegetables are tender-crisp.
- Add the cooked quinoa to the skillet and stir to combine.
- In a small bowl, whisk together the soy sauce and sesame oil. Pour the sauce over the quinoa and vegetables, and toss to coat evenly.
- Season with salt and pepper to taste.
- Cook for an additional 2-3 minutes until everything is heated through.
- Serve the quinoa and vegetable stir-fry hot, garnished with sesame seeds for an extra crunch.

Nutritional Information:

Calories: 250

Protein: 8g

Fat: 10g

Carbohydrates: 35g

Fiber: 6g

Baked Chicken Breast with Roasted Brussels Sprouts

Description: This wholesome meal features juicy baked chicken breast paired with roasted Brussels sprouts. It's a simple yet satisfying combination that will leave you feeling nourished and content.

Ingredients:

- 2 chicken breasts
- 2 cups Brussels sprouts, halved
- 2 tablespoons olive oil
- 2 cloves garlic, minced
- 1 teaspoon dried thyme
- Salt and pepper to taste
- Lemon wedges for serving

Instructions:

- Preheat the oven to 400°F (200°C).
- Season the chicken breasts with salt, pepper, and dried thyme on both sides.
- Heat olive oil in an oven-safe skillet over medium-high heat.

- Sear the chicken breasts for 2-3 minutes on each side until golden brown.
- Remove the chicken from the skillet and set aside.
- In the same skillet, add the halved Brussels sprouts, minced garlic, salt, and pepper. Toss to coat the Brussels sprouts in the oil and seasonings.
- Transfer the skillet to the preheated oven and bake for 15-20 minutes until the chicken is cooked through and the Brussels sprouts are tender and slightly caramelized.
- Remove from the oven and let the chicken rest for a few minutes.
- Serve the baked chicken breast alongside the roasted Brussels sprouts.
- Squeeze fresh lemon juice over the chicken and sprouts before enjoying.

Nutritional Information:

Calories: 320

Protein: 40g

Fat: 12g

Carbohydrates: 10g

Fiber: 4g

Lentil Soup with Spinach and Carrots

Description: Warm up with a comforting bowl of lentil

soup packed with nutritious spinach and carrots. This hearty soup is loaded with protein, fiber, and essential vitamins, making it a wholesome option for a satisfying meal.

Ingredients:

- 1 cup dried lentils, rinsed and drained
- 4 cups vegetable broth
- 1 onion, diced
- 2 carrots, diced
- 2 cloves garlic, minced
- 2 cups fresh spinach leaves
- 1 tablespoon olive oil
- 1 teaspoon cumin
- 1 teaspoon paprika
- Salt and pepper to taste

Instructions:

- Heat olive oil in a large pot over medium heat.
- Add the diced onion and minced garlic to the pot. Sauté for 2-3 minutes until the onion is translucent and fragrant.
- Add the diced carrots to the pot and cook for another 3-4 minutes.
- Stir in the rinsed lentils, cumin, paprika, salt, and pepper. Cook for 1-2 minutes to toast the spices.
- Pour in the vegetable broth and bring to a boil.
- Reduce the heat to low, cover the pot, and simmer for about 30-40 minutes until the lentils are tender.
- Add the fresh spinach leaves to the pot and cook

- for an additional 2-3 minutes until wilted.
- Adjust the seasoning if needed.
- Serve the lentil soup hot, and enjoy its nourishing goodness.

Nutritional Information:

Calories: 220

Protein: 15g

Fat: 4g

Carbohydrates: 35g

Fiber: 12g

Spinach Salad with Grilled Chicken and Avocado

Description: This refreshing spinach salad is a delightful blend of flavors and textures. It features grilled chicken, creamy avocado, and a tangy dressing that complements the freshness of the spinach leaves. It's a balanced and nutritious meal that will leave you feeling satisfied.

Ingredients:

- 2 cups fresh spinach leaves
- 1 grilled chicken breast, sliced
- 1 ripe avocado, sliced

- 1/4 cup cherry tomatoes, halved
- 2 tablespoons sliced almonds
- 2 tablespoons feta cheese

For the dressing:

- 2 tablespoons olive oil
- 1 tablespoon balsamic vinegar
- 1 teaspoon Dijon mustard
- Salt and pepper to taste

Instructions:

- In a large salad bowl, combine the fresh spinach leaves, sliced grilled chicken breast, avocado slices, cherry tomatoes, sliced almonds, and feta cheese.
- In a small bowl, whisk together the olive oil, balsamic vinegar, Dijon mustard, salt, and pepper to make the dressing.
- Drizzle the dressing over the spinach salad and toss gently to coat all the ingredients.
- Serve the spinach salad immediately, and enjoy the vibrant flavors and textures.

Nutritional Information:

Calories: 350

Protein: 25g

Fat: 22g

Carbohydrates: 15g

Fiber: 8g

Roasted Turkey Breast with Steamed Green Beans

Description: Indulge in the flavors of a succulent roasted turkey breast paired with tender steamed green beans. This wholesome and protein-packed meal is perfect for a hearty and satisfying dinner.

Ingredients:

- 1 turkey breast, boneless and skinless
- 2 cups fresh green beans
- 2 tablespoons olive oil
- 2 cloves garlic, minced
- 1 teaspoon dried rosemary
- Salt and pepper to taste
- Cranberry sauce for serving (optional)

Instructions:

- Preheat the oven to 375°F (190°C).
- Place the turkey breast in a roasting pan and season it with minced garlic, dried rosemary, salt, and pepper.
- Drizzle olive oil over the turkey breast, rubbing it all over the surface.
- Roast the turkey breast in the preheated oven for approximately 1 hour or until the internal temperature reaches 165°F (74°C).
- While the turkey is roasting, steam the green beans until they are crisp-tender, about 5-7

minutes.
- Once the turkey is cooked, remove it from the oven and let it rest for a few minutes before slicing.
- Serve the roasted turkey breast with steamed green beans.
- Accompany the meal with cranberry sauce for a burst of tangy sweetness, if desired.

Nutritional Information:

Calories: 300

Protein: 45g

Fat: 8g

Carbohydrates: 10g

Fiber: 4g

Brown Rice Bowl with Grilled Tofu and Mixed Vegetables

Description of the Meal: This Brown Rice Bowl with Grilled Tofu and Mixed Vegetables is a wholesome and satisfying dish that combines the nutty flavors of brown rice, the smokiness of grilled tofu, and a colorful assortment of mixed vegetables. It's a perfect choice for a nutritious and flavorful meal.

Ingredients:

- 1 cup brown rice
- 8 ounces firm tofu, drained and cubed
- 2 cups mixed vegetables (such as bell peppers, zucchini, and carrots), chopped
- 2 tablespoons soy sauce
- 1 tablespoon sesame oil
- 1 teaspoon garlic powder
- 1 teaspoon ginger powder
- Salt and pepper, to taste
- Fresh cilantro, for garnish

Instructions:

- Cook the brown rice according to the package instructions and set aside.
- Preheat a grill or grill pan over medium-high heat.
- In a bowl, combine the cubed tofu, soy sauce, sesame oil, garlic powder, ginger powder, salt, and pepper. Toss gently to coat the tofu evenly.
- Thread the marinated tofu and mixed vegetables onto skewers, alternating between them.
- Place the skewers on the preheated grill and cook for about 5 minutes per side, or until the tofu is lightly browned and the vegetables are tender.
- Remove the skewers from the grill and let them cool slightly.
- In serving bowls, divide the cooked brown rice, grilled tofu, and mixed vegetables.
- Garnish with fresh cilantro and serve hot.

Nutritional Information:

Calories: 350

Protein: 18g

Carbohydrates: 50g

Fat: 10g

Fiber: 8g

Shrimp and Vegetable Skewers with Brown Rice

Description of the Meal: Indulge in the delightful combination of succulent shrimp and vibrant vegetables with this Shrimp and Vegetable Skewers with Brown Rice dish. The skewers are grilled to perfection, infusing the ingredients with a smoky flavor that pairs wonderfully with the fluffy brown rice.

Ingredients:

- 1 pound shrimp, peeled and deveined
- 2 cups mixed vegetables (such as cherry tomatoes, bell peppers, and red onions), chopped
- 2 tablespoons olive oil
- 2 tablespoons lemon juice
- 1 teaspoon paprika
- 1 teaspoon dried oregano

- Salt and pepper, to taste
- Cooked brown rice, for serving

Instructions:

- Preheat the grill or grill pan over medium-high heat.
- In a bowl, combine the shrimp, mixed vegetables, olive oil, lemon juice, paprika, dried oregano, salt, and pepper. Toss gently to coat the ingredients evenly.
- Thread the marinated shrimp and vegetables onto skewers, alternating between them.
- Place the skewers on the preheated grill and cook for about 2-3 minutes per side, or until the shrimp turn pink and are cooked through.
- Remove the skewers from the grill and let them cool slightly.
- Serve the shrimp and vegetable skewers over a bed of cooked brown rice.

Nutritional Information:

Calories: 280

Protein: 25g

Carbohydrates: 20g

Fat: 10g

Fiber: 4g

Grilled Halibut with Asparagus and Quinoa

Description of the Meal: Experience the exquisite flavors of Grilled Halibut with Asparagus and Quinoa. The tender halibut fillets are lightly seasoned and grilled to perfection, while the asparagus adds a touch of freshness and the quinoa provides a satisfying and nutritious base.

Ingredients:

- 2 halibut fillets (6 ounces each)
- 1 bunch asparagus, trimmed
- 1 cup cooked quinoa
- 2 tablespoons lemon juice
- 2 tablespoons olive oil
- 1 teaspoon dried dill
- Salt and pepper, to taste
- Lemon wedges, for garnish

Instructions:

- Preheat the grill to medium heat.
- In a small bowl, combine the lemon juice, olive oil, dried dill, salt, and pepper.
- Brush the halibut fillets and asparagus with the marinade mixture.
- Place the halibut fillets and asparagus on the grill and cook for about 4-5 minutes per side, or until the fish is opaque and flakes easily with a fork.
- Remove the halibut and asparagus from the grill and let them cool slightly.

- In a serving dish, arrange the cooked quinoa and top it with the grilled halibut fillets and asparagus.
- Garnish with lemon wedges and serve warm.

Nutritional Information:

Calories: 350

Protein: 30g

Carbohydrates: 30g

Fat: 12g

Fiber: 6g

Vegetable Curry with Cauliflower Rice

Description of the Meal: Embrace the aromatic flavors of this Vegetable Curry with Cauliflower Rice. This vegan dish features a medley of colorful vegetables cooked in a rich and flavorful curry sauce, served over a bed of cauliflower rice for a low-carb twist.

Ingredients:

- 1 cauliflower head, grated or processed into rice-like consistency
- 2 cups mixed vegetables (such as broccoli, bell peppers, carrots, and peas), chopped

- 1 can (14 ounces) coconut milk
- 1 tablespoon curry powder
- 1 teaspoon turmeric
- 1 teaspoon cumin
- 1 teaspoon paprika
- 1 tablespoon olive oil
- Salt and pepper, to taste
- Fresh cilantro, for garnish

Instructions:

- Heat the olive oil in a large skillet over medium heat.
- Add the mixed vegetables to the skillet and sauté for 5 minutes until slightly tender.
- In a bowl, whisk together the coconut milk, curry powder, turmeric, cumin, paprika, salt, and pepper.
- Pour the coconut milk mixture over the sautéed vegetables and bring to a simmer.
- Reduce the heat to low and let the curry simmer for 10-15 minutes, allowing the flavors to meld together.
- Meanwhile, place the grated cauliflower in a microwave-safe bowl, cover, and microwave for 3-4 minutes until cooked.
- Fluff the cauliflower rice with a fork and divide it into serving bowls.
- Ladle the vegetable curry over the cauliflower rice.
- Garnish with fresh cilantro and serve hot.

Nutritional Information:

Calories: 250

Protein: 8g

Carbohydrates: 20g

Fat: 18g

Fiber: 8g

Baked Cod with Roasted Zucchini and Quinoa

Description of the Meal: Delight in the flavors of tender baked cod paired with roasted zucchini and fluffy quinoa in this wholesome and nutritious dish. The combination of succulent fish, caramelized zucchini, and nutty quinoa creates a satisfying and well-rounded meal.

Ingredients:

- 2 cod fillets (6 ounces each)
- 2 zucchini, sliced
- 1 cup cooked quinoa
- 2 tablespoons lemon juice
- 2 tablespoons olive oil
- 1 teaspoon dried thyme
- Salt and pepper, to taste
- Fresh parsley, for garnish

Instructions:

- Preheat the oven to 375°F (190°C).
- Place the cod fillets in a baking dish and drizzle

with lemon juice and olive oil.
- Season the cod with dried thyme, salt, and pepper.
- Arrange the sliced zucchini around the cod fillets.
- Bake in the preheated oven for 15-20 minutes or until the cod is cooked through and flakes easily with a fork.
- While the cod is baking, cook the quinoa according to package instructions.
- Once cooked, fluff the quinoa with a fork.
- Remove the baked cod and roasted zucchini from the oven.
- Serve the cod fillets over a bed of cooked quinoa.
- Garnish with fresh parsley and serve hot.

Nutritional Information:

Calories: 300

Protein: 30g

Carbohydrates: 25g

Fat: 10g

Fiber: 6g

Chicken and Vegetable Stir-Fry with Brown Rice

Description of the Meal: Indulge in the vibrant flavors of this Chicken and Vegetable Stir-Fry with Brown Rice. Tender chicken, crisp vegetables, and aromatic stir-fry sauce come together in a satisfying dish that is both nutritious and delicious.

Ingredients:

- 2 boneless, skinless chicken breasts, thinly sliced
- 2 cups mixed vegetables (such as bell peppers, broccoli, and snap peas), sliced
- 2 tablespoons soy sauce
- 1 tablespoon hoisin sauce
- 1 tablespoon sesame oil
- 1 teaspoon minced garlic
- 1 teaspoon minced ginger
- 2 cups cooked brown rice
- Green onions, for garnish
- Sesame seeds, for garnish

Instructions:

- Heat sesame oil in a large skillet or wok over medium-high heat.
- Add the sliced chicken to the skillet and cook until browned and cooked through.
- Remove the chicken from the skillet and set aside.
- In the same skillet, add the mixed vegetables and stir-fry for 3-4 minutes until crisp-tender.
- In a small bowl, whisk together soy sauce, hoisin sauce, minced garlic, and minced ginger.
- Pour the sauce mixture over the vegetables in the skillet.
- Return the cooked chicken to the skillet and toss to coat everything in the sauce.
- Cook for an additional 2-3 minutes to heat through.

- Divide the cooked brown rice among serving plates.
- Top the rice with the chicken and vegetable stir-fry.
- Garnish with sliced green onions and sesame seeds.
- Serve hot.

Nutritional Information:

Calories: 400

Protein: 30g

Carbohydrates: 45g

Fat: 12g

Fiber: 8g

Spinach and Mushroom Omelette with Whole Grain Toast

Description of the Meal: Enjoy a nutritious and flavorful breakfast with this Spinach and Mushroom Omelette paired with whole grain toast. The fluffy omelette filled with sautéed spinach and mushrooms provides a satisfying and protein-packed start to your day.

Ingredients:

- 3 large eggs
- 1 cup spinach, chopped
- ½ cup mushrooms, sliced
- 2 tablespoons diced onions
- 1 tablespoon olive oil
- Salt and pepper, to taste
- 2 slices whole grain toast

Instructions:

- In a bowl, whisk the eggs until well beaten. Set aside.
- Heat the olive oil in a non-stick skillet over medium heat.
- Add the diced onions and sauté until translucent.
- Add the sliced mushrooms to the skillet and cook until they start to brown.
- Add the chopped spinach to the skillet and cook until wilted.
- Season the vegetables with salt and pepper to taste.
- Pour the beaten eggs over the sautéed vegetables in the skillet.
- Gently swirl the skillet to distribute the eggs and vegetables evenly.
- Cook the omelette for about 2-3 minutes until the edges start to set.
- Carefully fold the omelette in half using a spatula.
- Continue cooking for an additional 1-2 minutes until the omelette is cooked through.
- Toast the whole grain bread slices until golden.
- Serve the spinach and mushroom omelette alongside the whole grain toast.
- Enjoy while warm.

Nutritional Information:

Calories: 320

Protein: 18g

Carbohydrates: 22g

Fat: 18g

Fiber: 6g

Grilled Steak with Roasted Sweet Potatoes and Broccoli

Description of the Meal: Savor the hearty flavors of Grilled Steak with Roasted Sweet Potatoes and Broccoli. The tender and juicy steak pairs perfectly with the caramelized sweetness of roasted sweet potatoes and the vibrant greenness of broccoli, creating a balanced and satisfying meal.

Ingredients:

- 2 steak cuts (such as ribeye or sirloin)
- 2 medium sweet potatoes, peeled and cubed
- 2 cups broccoli florets
- 2 tablespoons olive oil
- 1 teaspoon garlic powder

- 1 teaspoon dried rosemary
- Salt and pepper, to taste

Instructions:

- Preheat the grill to medium-high heat.
- Brush the steaks with olive oil and season them with garlic powder, dried rosemary, salt, and pepper.
- Place the seasoned steaks on the preheated grill and cook for 4-6 minutes per side, or until desired doneness is reached.
- Remove the steaks from the grill and let them rest for a few minutes before slicing.
- While the steaks are resting, preheat the oven to 400°F (200°C).
- In a bowl, toss the cubed sweet potatoes with olive oil, salt, and pepper.
- Spread the sweet potatoes in a single layer on a baking sheet and roast in the preheated oven for 25-30 minutes, or until they are tender and golden.
- In another bowl, toss the broccoli florets with olive oil, salt, and pepper.
- Add the broccoli to the same baking sheet with the sweet potatoes and roast for an additional 10-12 minutes, or until the broccoli is crisp-tender.
- Slice the grilled steaks against the grain into thin strips.
- Serve the sliced steak alongside the roasted sweet potatoes and broccoli.
- Enjoy while hot.

Nutritional Information:

Calories: 450

Protein: 35g

Carbohydrates: 35g

Fat: 20g

Fiber: 8g

Quinoa Salad with Roasted Vegetables and Chickpeas

Description of the Meal: Indulge in the wholesome goodness of Quinoa Salad with Roasted Vegetables and Chickpeas. This vibrant and nutritious salad combines fluffy quinoa with a medley of roasted vegetables and protein-packed chickpeas, creating a satisfying and flavorful dish.

Ingredients:

- 1 cup cooked quinoa
- 2 cups mixed vegetables (such as bell peppers, zucchini, and eggplant), diced
- 1 can (14 ounces) chickpeas, drained and rinsed
- 2 tablespoons olive oil
- 1 teaspoon dried herbs (such as thyme or rosemary)

- Salt and pepper, to taste
- Lemon vinaigrette dressing (store-bought or homemade)

Instructions:

- Preheat the oven to 425°F (220°C).
- In a mixing bowl, combine the diced mixed vegetables, chickpeas, olive oil, dried herbs, salt, and pepper. Toss until the vegetables and chickpeas are well coated.
- Spread the vegetable and chickpea mixture in a single layer on a baking sheet.
- Roast in the preheated oven for 20-25 minutes, or until the vegetables are tender and slightly caramelized.
- In a large serving bowl, combine the cooked quinoa with the roasted vegetables and chickpeas.
- Drizzle the lemon vinaigrette dressing over the salad and toss to combine.
- Adjust the seasoning with additional salt and pepper, if desired.
- Serve the quinoa salad at room temperature or chilled.

Nutritional Information:

Calories: 350

Protein: 12g

Carbohydrates: 45g

Fat: 14g

Fiber: 10g

Turkey Chili with Beans and Mixed Greens

Description of the Meal: Warm up with a hearty bowl of Turkey Chili with Beans and Mixed Greens. This flavorful and nutritious chili features lean ground turkey, a variety of beans, and a generous serving of mixed greens for added freshness and vitamins.

Ingredients:

- 1 pound lean ground turkey
- 1 can (14 ounces) diced tomatoes
- 1 can (14 ounces) kidney beans, drained and rinsed
- 1 can (14 ounces) black beans, drained and rinsed
- 1 cup mixed greens (such as spinach or kale), chopped
- 1 onion, diced
- 2 cloves garlic, minced
- 1 tablespoon chili powder
- 1 teaspoon cumin
- ½ teaspoon paprika
- Salt and pepper, to taste
- Fresh cilantro, for garnish

Instructions:

- In a large pot or Dutch oven, cook the ground turkey over medium heat until browned.

- Add the diced onion and minced garlic to the pot and sauté until the onion is translucent.
- Stir in the chili powder, cumin, paprika, salt, and pepper, and cook for another minute to toast the spices.
- Add the diced tomatoes, kidney beans, and black beans to the pot, along with a cup of water.
- Bring the chili to a simmer and let it cook for 20-25 minutes, allowing the flavors to meld together.
- Add the chopped mixed greens to the pot and cook for an additional 5 minutes until wilted.
- Adjust the seasoning with additional salt and pepper, if needed.
- Ladle the turkey chili into bowls and garnish with fresh cilantro.
- Serve hot.

Nutritional Information:

Calories: 400

Protein: 30g

Carbohydrates: 40g

Fat: 10g

Fiber: 12g

Baked Cod with Steamed Asparagus

and Brown Rice

Description of the Meal: Delight in the delicate flavors of Baked Cod with Steamed Asparagus and Brown Rice. The tender cod fillets are baked to perfection, accompanied by vibrant green asparagus and nutty brown rice, creating a balanced and nourishing dish.

Ingredients:

- 2 cod fillets (6 ounces each)
- 1 bunch asparagus, trimmed
- 1 cup cooked brown rice
- 2 tablespoons lemon juice
- 2 tablespoons olive oil
- 1 teaspoon dried dill
- Salt and pepper, to taste
- Lemon wedges, for serving

Instructions:

- Preheat the oven to 375°F (190°C).
- Place the cod fillets in a baking dish and drizzle with lemon juice and olive oil.
- Season the cod with dried dill, salt, and pepper.
- Arrange the trimmed asparagus around the cod fillets.
- Bake in the preheated oven for 15-20 minutes or until the cod is cooked through and flakes easily with a fork.
- While the cod is baking, steam the asparagus until crisp-tender, about 5-7 minutes.

- Once cooked, fluff the brown rice with a fork.
- Remove the baked cod and steamed asparagus from the oven and steamer, respectively.
- Serve the cod fillets over a bed of cooked brown rice and alongside the steamed asparagus.
- Garnish with lemon wedges and serve hot.

Nutritional Information:

Calories: 350

Protein: 30g

Carbohydrates: 30g

Fat: 12g

Fiber: 6g

Vegetable and Lentil Curry with Quinoa

Description of the Meal: Enjoy the rich and aromatic flavors of Vegetable and Lentil Curry with Quinoa. This hearty and nutritious curry features a medley of colorful vegetables, protein-packed lentils, and fluffy quinoa, making it a satisfying and wholesome meal.

Ingredients:

- 1 cup cooked quinoa
- 1 cup lentils, cooked

- 2 cups mixed vegetables (such as carrots, bell peppers, and peas), diced
- 1 onion, diced
- 2 cloves garlic, minced
- 1 can (14 ounces) coconut milk
- 2 tablespoons curry powder
- 1 teaspoon cumin
- 1 teaspoon turmeric
- Salt and pepper, to taste
- Fresh cilantro, for garnish

Instructions:

- In a large skillet or pot, sauté the diced onion and minced garlic until fragrant and translucent.
- Add the diced mixed vegetables to the skillet and cook for a few minutes until slightly softened.
- Stir in the curry powder, cumin, turmeric, salt, and pepper, and cook for another minute to toast the spices.
- Pour in the coconut milk and bring the mixture to a simmer.
- Add the cooked lentils to the skillet and stir to combine.
- Let the curry simmer for 10-15 minutes to allow the flavors to meld together and the vegetables to become tender.
- Adjust the seasoning with additional salt and pepper, if desired.
- Serve the vegetable and lentil curry over a bed of cooked quinoa.
- Garnish with fresh cilantro.
- Enjoy while hot.

Nutritional Information:

Calories: 380

Protein: 18g

Carbohydrates: 50g

Fat: 15g

Fiber: 12g

Grilled Chicken Breast with Steamed Cauliflower and Brown Rice

Description of the Meal: Enjoy a satisfying and healthy meal with Grilled Chicken Breast, Steamed Cauliflower, and Brown Rice. The tender and flavorful grilled chicken is paired with nutritious steamed cauliflower and wholesome brown rice, creating a balanced and nourishing dish.

Ingredients:

- 2 chicken breasts
- 1 small head of cauliflower, cut into florets
- 1 cup cooked brown rice
- 2 tablespoons olive oil
- 1 teaspoon garlic powder
- Salt and pepper, to taste

Instructions:

- Preheat the grill to medium-high heat.
- Season the chicken breasts with olive oil, garlic powder, salt, and pepper.
- Place the seasoned chicken breasts on the preheated grill and cook for 6-8 minutes per side, or until the internal temperature reaches 165°F (74°C).
- While the chicken is grilling, steam the cauliflower florets until tender, about 5-7 minutes.
- Cook the brown rice according to package instructions.
- Once the chicken is cooked, remove it from the grill and let it rest for a few minutes before slicing.
- Serve the grilled chicken breast alongside steamed cauliflower and a serving of cooked brown rice.
- Enjoy while hot.

Nutritional Information:

Calories: 400

Protein: 35g

Carbohydrates: 30g

Fat: 15g

Fiber: 6g

Roasted Salmon with Lemon-Dill Sauce and Steamed Spinach

Description of the Meal: Indulge in the succulent flavors of Roasted Salmon with Lemon-Dill Sauce and Steamed Spinach. The perfectly roasted salmon fillets are complemented by a tangy lemon-dill sauce and a side of nutritious steamed spinach, creating a delicious and wholesome dish.

Ingredients:

- 2 salmon fillets (6 ounces each)
- 2 tablespoons fresh lemon juice
- 1 tablespoon olive oil
- 1 tablespoon fresh dill, chopped
- Salt and pepper, to taste
- 1 cup fresh spinach

Instructions:

- Preheat the oven to 400°F (200°C).
- Place the salmon fillets on a baking sheet lined with parchment paper.
- Drizzle the salmon with fresh lemon juice and olive oil.
- Season the salmon with fresh dill, salt, and pepper.
- Roast the salmon in the preheated oven for 12-15 minutes, or until the fish is cooked through and flakes easily with a fork.

- While the salmon is roasting, steam the fresh spinach until wilted, about 2-3 minutes.
- Once cooked, remove the salmon from the oven and let it rest for a few minutes.
- Serve the roasted salmon fillets alongside steamed spinach.
- Drizzle the salmon with any remaining lemon juice and olive oil from the baking sheet.
- Enjoy while hot.

Nutritional Information:

Calories: 350

Protein: 30g

Carbohydrates: 5g

Fat: 22g

Fiber: 2g

Stir-Fried Shrimp with Mixed Vegetables and Brown Rice Noodles

Description of the Meal: Delight in the flavors of Stir-Fried Shrimp with Mixed Vegetables and Brown Rice Noodles. This vibrant and nutritious dish features succulent shrimp, a colorful array of mixed vegetables, and tender brown rice noodles, creating a satisfying and flavorful meal.

Ingredients:

- 1 pound shrimp, peeled and deveined
- 8 ounces brown rice noodles
- 2 cups mixed vegetables (such as bell peppers, broccoli, and carrots), sliced
- 2 tablespoons soy sauce
- 1 tablespoon sesame oil
- 1 tablespoon honey
- 1 teaspoon ginger, minced
- 2 cloves garlic, minced
- Salt and pepper, to taste

Instructions:

- Cook the brown rice noodles according to package instructions. Drain and set aside.
- In a small bowl, whisk together the soy sauce, sesame oil, honey, ginger, garlic, salt, and pepper to make the sauce.
- Heat a large skillet or wok over medium-high heat and add a tablespoon of oil.
- Add the shrimp to the skillet and stir-fry for 2-3 minutes, or until they turn pink and opaque. Remove the shrimp from the skillet and set aside.
- In the same skillet, add the mixed vegetables and stir-fry for 3-4 minutes, or until they are crisp-tender.
- Return the shrimp to the skillet and add the cooked brown rice noodles.
- Pour the sauce over the shrimp, vegetables, and noodles, and stir to coat everything evenly.

- Cook for an additional 1-2 minutes, until everything is heated through.
- Adjust the seasoning with additional salt and pepper, if desired.
- Serve the stir-fried shrimp, mixed vegetables, and brown rice noodles hot.

Nutritional Information:

Calories: 400

Protein: 25g

Carbohydrates: 55g

Fat: 10g

Fiber: 6g

Grilled Tofu and Vegetable Skewers with Quinoa

Description of the Meal: Experience a delightful combination of flavors with Grilled Tofu and Vegetable Skewers served with Quinoa. These colorful and protein-packed skewers feature marinated tofu and a variety of grilled vegetables, accompanied by fluffy quinoa for a satisfying and nutritious meal.

Ingredients:

- 1 block of tofu, cut into cubes
- 1 red bell pepper, cut into chunks
- 1 zucchini, sliced
- 1 red onion, cut into chunks
- 1 cup cooked quinoa
- 2 tablespoons soy sauce
- 1 tablespoon olive oil
- 1 tablespoon maple syrup
- 1 teaspoon garlic powder
- Salt and pepper, to taste

Instructions:

- Preheat the grill to medium heat.
- In a bowl, whisk together the soy sauce, olive oil, maple syrup, garlic powder, salt, and pepper to make the marinade.
- Thread the tofu cubes, red bell pepper chunks, zucchini slices, and red onion chunks onto skewers, alternating the ingredients.
- Brush the marinade over the tofu and vegetable skewers, making sure they are evenly coated.
- Place the skewers on the preheated grill and cook for about 10 minutes, turning occasionally, until the tofu is lightly browned and the vegetables are tender.
- While the skewers are grilling, cook the quinoa according to package instructions.
- Once cooked, fluff the quinoa with a fork.
- Serve the grilled tofu and vegetable skewers alongside a serving of cooked quinoa.
- Enjoy while hot.

Nutritional Information:

Calories: 350

Protein: 20g

Carbohydrates: 40g

Fat: 15g

Fiber: 6g

Turkey Meatballs with Whole Wheat Pasta and Marinara Sauce

Description of the Meal: Indulge in the comforting flavors of Turkey Meatballs with Whole Wheat Pasta and Marinara Sauce. These tender and flavorful turkey meatballs are paired with whole wheat pasta and a rich marinara sauce, creating a satisfying and wholesome dish.

Ingredients:

- 1 pound ground turkey
- 1/4 cup breadcrumbs
- 1/4 cup grated Parmesan cheese
- 1/4 cup chopped fresh parsley
- 1 egg, beaten
- 2 cloves garlic, minced
- 1 teaspoon dried oregano
- 1/2 teaspoon salt
- 1/4 teaspoon black pepper

- 8 ounces whole wheat pasta
- 2 cups marinara sauce
- Fresh basil, for garnish

Instructions:

- In a large bowl, combine the ground turkey, breadcrumbs, Parmesan cheese, chopped parsley, beaten egg, minced garlic, dried oregano, salt, and black pepper. Mix well until all ingredients are evenly incorporated.
- Shape the mixture into meatballs, about 1 inch in diameter.
- In a large skillet, heat a tablespoon of olive oil over medium heat.
- Add the turkey meatballs to the skillet and cook for 8-10 minutes, or until browned and cooked through. Make sure to turn the meatballs occasionally for even cooking.
- While the meatballs are cooking, cook the whole wheat pasta according to package instructions. Drain and set aside.
- In a separate saucepan, heat the marinara sauce over low heat until warmed through.
- Add the cooked meatballs to the marinara sauce and simmer for a few minutes to allow the flavors to blend together.
- Serve the turkey meatballs and marinara sauce over a bed of cooked whole wheat pasta.
- Garnish with fresh basil leaves.
- Enjoy while hot.

Nutritional Information:

Calories: 400

Protein: 25g

Carbohydrates: 40g

Fat: 15g

Fiber: 6g

Broccoli and Mushroom Frittata with Whole Grain Toast

Description of the Meal: Start your day with a nutritious and flavorful Broccoli and Mushroom Frittata paired with Whole Grain Toast. This hearty and protein-packed frittata features tender broccoli florets, earthy mushrooms, and fluffy eggs, providing a satisfying and energizing breakfast.

Ingredients:

- 6 large eggs
- 1 cup broccoli florets, blanched and chopped
- 1 cup sliced mushrooms
- 1/2 cup shredded cheddar cheese
- 1/4 cup chopped green onions
- 1 tablespoon olive oil
- Salt and pepper, to taste
- Whole grain toast, for serving

Instructions:

- Preheat the oven to 375°F (190°C).
- In a bowl, whisk the eggs until well beaten. Season with salt and pepper.
- Heat the olive oil in an oven-safe skillet over medium heat.
- Add the sliced mushrooms and sauté until they release their moisture and become tender, about 5 minutes.
- Add the blanched and chopped broccoli florets to the skillet and cook for another 2 minutes.
- Pour the beaten eggs into the skillet, making sure they cover the vegetables evenly.
- Sprinkle the shredded cheddar cheese and chopped green onions over the egg mixture.
- Cook on the stovetop for 2-3 minutes, or until the edges of the frittata start to set.
- Transfer the skillet to the preheated oven and bake for 10-12 minutes, or until the frittata is set and lightly golden on top.
- Remove from the oven and let it cool for a few minutes.
- Cut the frittata into wedges and serve with whole grain toast.
- Enjoy as a delicious breakfast or brunch option.

Nutritional Information:

Calories: 250

Protein: 16g

Carbohydrates: 10g

Fat: 16g

Fiber: 2g

Quinoa Bowl with Roasted Chicken, Avocado, and Mixed Greens

Description of the Meal: Savor the flavors of a nutritious Quinoa Bowl with Roasted Chicken, Avocado, and Mixed Greens. This vibrant and protein-rich bowl features fluffy quinoa, tender roasted chicken, creamy avocado, and a medley of fresh mixed greens, creating a filling and wholesome meal.

Ingredients:

- 1 cup cooked quinoa
- 1 cup roasted chicken breast, shredded
- 1 avocado, sliced
- 2 cups mixed greens
- 1/4 cup cherry tomatoes, halved
- 1/4 cup cucumber, sliced
- 2 tablespoons lemon juice
- 1 tablespoon olive oil
- Salt and pepper, to taste

Instructions:

- In a bowl, combine the cooked quinoa, shredded roasted chicken breast, mixed greens, cherry

tomatoes, and cucumber.
- In a small separate bowl, whisk together the lemon juice, olive oil, salt, and pepper to make the dressing.
- Drizzle the dressing over the quinoa mixture and toss to coat everything evenly.
- Arrange the sliced avocado on top of the quinoa bowl.
- Season with additional salt and pepper, if desired.
- Enjoy the quinoa bowl as a light and refreshing meal.

Nutritional Information:

Calories: 400

Protein: 30g

Carbohydrates: 30g

Fat: 20g

Fiber: 8g

CONCLUSION

In conclusion, this book on breast cancer diet serves as a comprehensive guide, empowering individuals with knowledge and practical strategies to optimize their nutritional choices in the face of breast cancer. By emphasizing the importance of a well-balanced diet, rich in whole foods, antioxidants, and anti-inflammatory compounds, readers are equipped with the tools to support their overall health and potentially enhance their treatment outcomes. Through the exploration of evidence-based research and expert insights, this book has shed light on the significant role that nutrition plays in the prevention, management, and recovery from breast cancer. By making informed dietary decisions, individuals can take an active role in their well-being, fostering a sense of empowerment and hope. As we move forward, let us remember that each meal is an opportunity to nourish both body and spirit, and through the choices we make, we can strive for a healthier future, empowering ourselves and inspiring others on the journey towards wellness.